MW01170094

VIAGRA (SILDENAFIL) MEN'S GUIDE:

Fast Solutions for Erectile Dysfunction and Lasting Satisfaction

David Bennett

Introduction

What is Viagra (Sildenafil)?
Viagra (Sildenafil) is one of the most well-known medications for the treatment of erectile dysfunction (ED), approved by the FDA in 1998. Since its introduction, Viagra has helped millions of men worldwide overcome sexual performance issues and regain confidence in their intimate relationships. Originally developed as a heart medication, its powerful effect on enhancing blood flow to the penis was soon recognized as a breakthrough in treating ED. This discovery changed the way men with ED could manage their condition, offering a safe and effective solution.

Viagra works by inhibiting an enzyme called PDE-5, which regulates blood flow in the penis. By increasing the blood flow to the erectile tissues, Viagra helps men achieve and maintain a strong and lasting erection when sexually stimulated. It has become the go-to medication for men of various ages, offering a reliable solution to the challenges of erectile dysfunction.

Why this Guide?

This guide is designed to provide comprehensive information about Viagra (Sildenafil) and how it can positively impact your sexual health and overall well-being. Whether you're new to Viagra or simply looking for detailed insights into how it works, this book aims to educate and empower you to take control of your sexual performance and confidence.

In this guide, we will walk you through:

- The causes of erectile dysfunction and how it can affect your life.
- How Viagra works to treat ED and improve your sexual performance.
- The benefits, safety considerations, and potential side effects of Viagra.
- Real-life success stories of men who have used Viagra to improve their intimacy and relationships.

Take Control of Your Sexual Health

Erectile dysfunction can be a frustrating and emotionally challenging condition, but it doesn't have to define you. With the help of Viagra, men around the world have reclaimed their vitality and confidence in the bedroom. This guide will equip you with the knowledge to make informed decisions about your sexual health and understand how Viagra can work for you.

It's time to break free from the limitations of erectile dysfunction and rediscover the passion and connection in your intimate relationships. Viagra offers you the opportunity to perform at your best and feel confident in your abilities, allowing you to experience a renewed sense of sexual fulfillment.

Let's begin your journey to better sexual health and satisfaction.

Chapter 1: Understanding Erectile Dysfunction (ED) and Its Impact on Life

Erectile dysfunction (ED) is a common sexual health issue that affects millions of men worldwide. It is defined as the persistent inability to achieve or maintain an erection firm enough for satisfactory sexual intercourse. While occasional difficulties with erections can occur due to fatigue, stress, or alcohol consumption, ED is diagnosed when this issue becomes a frequent and ongoing challenge.

What Causes Erectile Dysfunction?

ED can be caused by a variety of factors, and these can generally be categorized into two main groups: physical and psychological causes. Many men may experience ED as a result of a combination of these factors.

- **Physical Causes**:
  - **Cardiovascular disease**: Conditions such as high blood pressure, atherosclerosis (hardening of the arteries), and heart disease can restrict blood flow to the penis, making it difficult to achieve an erection.
  - **Diabetes**: This condition can damage the blood vessels and nerves responsible for erections, leading to ED.

- o **Obesity**: Being overweight is linked to various health issues, including heart disease and diabetes, which can cause ED.
- o **Hormonal Imbalances**: Low levels of testosterone or other hormonal imbalances can affect sexual performance.
- o **Neurological Disorders**: Conditions like Parkinson's disease, multiple sclerosis, or spinal cord injuries can disrupt the signals between the brain and the body necessary for an erection.
- o **Medications**: Certain medications, including antidepressants, blood pressure drugs, and treatments for prostate conditions, can interfere with erectile function.
- o **Smoking, Alcohol, and Drug Use**: These substances can affect blood flow and nerve function, contributing to ED.
- **Psychological Causes**:
  - o **Stress**: Both work-related and personal stress can affect your ability to perform sexually.
  - o **Anxiety**: Performance anxiety, or the fear of not being able to satisfy your partner, can actually prevent you from achieving an erection.

- **Depression**: Mental health issues like depression can lower libido and make it harder to become sexually aroused.
- **Relationship Problems**: Emotional distance or unresolved conflicts with your partner can result in decreased sexual interest and performance issues.

In many cases, ED may be a symptom of an underlying health condition. For instance, it could be the first sign of cardiovascular disease, signaling a problem with blood circulation. This is why it's essential to address ED not just as a sexual problem but as a potential indicator of other health concerns.

The Emotional Impact of Erectile Dysfunction

The effects of ED extend beyond the physical symptoms. For many men, the inability to achieve or maintain an erection can lead to feelings of inadequacy, frustration, and embarrassment. Over time, this can affect a man's self-esteem and lead to more significant emotional and psychological challenges, including:

- **Loss of Confidence**: When ED becomes a regular issue, many men begin to doubt their ability to perform sexually, which can lead to avoiding intimate situations altogether.

- **Strained Relationships**: Sexual intimacy is a crucial part of most romantic relationships. ED can create tension between partners, especially if it leads to reduced communication or feelings of rejection.
- **Depression and Anxiety**: ED can contribute to mental health issues, including depression and anxiety, particularly when it significantly impacts a man's self-image or his relationship with his partner.
- **Avoidance of Intimacy**: Many men experiencing ED may withdraw from intimate encounters, fearing repeated failure, which can further isolate them and lead to greater emotional distress.

ED is More Common Than You Think

It's important to recognize that erectile dysfunction is a widespread condition that affects men of all ages. While the likelihood of experiencing ED increases with age, it is not exclusive to older men. Factors like stress, anxiety, and lifestyle choices mean that men in their 20s, 30s, and 40s can also experience ED.

Studies show that nearly 30 million men in the United States alone are affected by ED, and the numbers are growing as more men seek treatment and become open about their struggles. Despite its prevalence, many men feel uncomfortable discussing ED, either with their partners or with healthcare professionals. This reluctance can delay treatment and prolong the emotional and physical strain caused by the condition.

Treatment Options for Erectile Dysfunction

There are many ways to address erectile dysfunction, ranging from lifestyle changes and psychological support to medical treatments. Some common approaches include:

- **Lifestyle Changes**: Adopting a healthier lifestyle can significantly improve erectile function. This includes quitting smoking, reducing alcohol intake, losing weight, and getting regular exercise to improve blood circulation.
- **Psychological Counseling**: For men whose ED is linked to psychological issues, therapy or counseling can help address the underlying causes of anxiety, stress, or relationship problems.

- **Medication**: Oral medications like Viagra (Sildenafil) are one of the most popular and effective treatments for ED. These drugs work by increasing blood flow to the penis, making it easier to achieve and maintain an erection during sexual arousal. Viagra is particularly effective because it can be taken as needed, offering men a flexible and reliable solution to their ED.
- **Other Treatments**: In some cases, men may require other treatments such as hormone therapy, penile injections, vacuum devices, or even surgery. The appropriate treatment depends on the individual's health and the severity of their ED.

The Importance of Seeking Help

If you or your partner is experiencing ED, it's crucial to seek help from a healthcare provider. ED is not something that should be ignored or left untreated. Aside from improving sexual performance, addressing ED can also enhance your overall health and well-being.

Open communication with your partner about ED is equally important. Many men struggle silently with the condition, which can worsen the emotional toll. By talking openly about ED and exploring treatment options together, you can strengthen your relationship and ensure that both partners feel supported.

Chapter 2: How Viagra Works

Viagra (Sildenafil) is one of the most trusted medications for treating erectile dysfunction (ED) due to its proven effectiveness and safety profile. Understanding how Viagra works can help you feel more confident about its use and know what to expect when taking it. This chapter will explain the science behind Viagra, how it affects your body, and why it's a reliable solution for millions of men worldwide.

The Science Behind Viagra (Sildenafil)

Viagra's active ingredient, Sildenafil, belongs to a class of drugs called **phosphodiesterase type 5 (PDE-5) inhibitors**. To understand how it works, let's break down the natural process of achieving an erection and how ED disrupts it.

- **The Erection Process**: When a man is sexually aroused, the brain sends signals to the blood vessels in the penis, causing them to widen and allow more blood to flow into the erectile tissues. This increased blood flow is what causes the penis to become firm and erect. The process is controlled by the release of a chemical called **nitric oxide**, which helps relax the smooth muscles in the blood vessels, allowing them to expand.

- **The Role of PDE-5**: After sexual stimulation and erection, the body produces an enzyme called **PDE-5**. This enzyme breaks down another chemical called **cyclic guanosine monophosphate (cGMP),** which is responsible for regulating blood flow to the penis. When PDE-5 breaks down cGMP, the blood vessels constrict, and the erection ends.
- **How ED Affects the Process**: In men with ED, the release of nitric oxide may be insufficient, or the action of PDE-5 may be too strong, leading to the inability to achieve or maintain an erection. The balance between blood flow into the penis and the chemical signals that relax the blood vessels is disrupted, resulting in erectile difficulties.

How Viagra Helps

Viagra works by inhibiting the action of PDE-5, preventing it from breaking down cGMP too quickly. By doing so, it allows the blood vessels in the penis to remain dilated longer, ensuring sufficient blood flow to achieve and maintain an erection during sexual stimulation.

- **Boosts cGMP Levels**: By blocking PDE-5, Viagra helps maintain higher levels of cGMP in the body. This results in the smooth muscles of the penis staying relaxed for longer, which promotes sustained blood flow and a firm erection.

- **Requires Sexual Stimulation**: It's important to note that Viagra doesn't cause an erection on its own. Sexual arousal is still necessary to trigger the release of nitric oxide and the subsequent chain of events that lead to an erection. Viagra simply supports this process by enhancing the body's natural ability to achieve an erection when sexually stimulated.
- **Time to Action**: Typically, Viagra takes effect within 30 to 60 minutes after ingestion, though some men may experience results sooner. The medication works best when taken on an empty stomach, as a large or high-fat meal can delay its absorption. Once in effect, Viagra can help a man achieve an erection for up to four to five hours, though this doesn't mean an erection will last the entire time. It simply means the body remains more responsive to sexual arousal during this window.

Viagra's Effectiveness

Clinical studies have shown that Viagra is highly effective in treating erectile dysfunction across a wide range of causes, including physical, psychological, and age-related factors. It has been proven to help about **70-85% of men** achieve improved erections, making it one of the most successful treatments for ED.

- **Age**: Viagra is effective for men of various age groups, including older men who may experience ED as a result of age-related health issues.
- **Underlying Health Conditions**: Men with chronic conditions like diabetes, high blood pressure, or cardiovascular diseases have also experienced significant improvements in erectile function after taking Viagra.
- **Mental Health and ED**: Men whose ED is related to anxiety or stress may also benefit from Viagra. By improving their physical ability to achieve an erection, many men find that their confidence in sexual situations increases, which helps reduce the psychological barriers associated with ED.

How Long Does Viagra Last?

The effects of Viagra can last for several hours, allowing flexibility in terms of sexual activity. However, Viagra's effectiveness gradually diminishes as it is metabolized by the body, and factors like age, liver function, and general health can influence how long it remains active.

- **Average Duration**: Most men will find that the effects last between **four and five hours**. During this period, you may be able to achieve multiple erections if you are sexually aroused again after ejaculation.

- **Extended Effect in Some Cases**: For some men, Viagra may continue to provide mild effects for up to 6 hours, but this varies from person to person. If you still have an erection after four hours without sexual stimulation, this could indicate a condition called **priapism**, which requires immediate medical attention.

What to Expect When Taking Viagra

For men using Viagra for the first time, knowing what to expect can help you make the most of its benefits. Here are some key points to keep in mind:

- **Optimal Use**: Viagra should be taken about 30 to 60 minutes before sexual activity. It is important to plan accordingly, especially if you are coordinating intimate moments with your partner.
- **Diet Considerations**: As mentioned earlier, taking Viagra on an empty stomach or with a light meal will ensure faster absorption and more predictable effects. A heavy or high-fat meal may delay its onset by up to an hour or more.
- **Alcohol**: Drinking large amounts of alcohol before taking Viagra can reduce its effectiveness, as alcohol can impair your ability to achieve an erection. It's best to limit alcohol consumption when using Viagra for optimal results.

- **Side Effects**: While Viagra is generally well-tolerated, some men may experience mild side effects such as headaches, flushing, nasal congestion, dizziness, or indigestion. These side effects are typically temporary and subside as the medication wears off. If side effects persist or worsen, it's important to consult with a healthcare professional.

When Viagra Might Not Work

Though Viagra is highly effective, it may not work for everyone on the first try. There are a few reasons why this might happen:

- **Incorrect Timing**: If you don't wait long enough after taking Viagra, or if you take it too long before sexual activity, it may not be fully effective. Be sure to follow the recommended timing for use.
- **Insufficient Stimulation**: Remember, Viagra requires sexual stimulation to work. If there is not enough arousal, the medication will not have its desired effect.
- **Underlying Health Conditions**: In some cases, ED may be caused by severe physical conditions that Viagra cannot fully address. If Viagra doesn't work after a few tries, it's a good idea to talk to your doctor about adjusting the dose or exploring other treatment options.

Viagra's Proven Track Record

Since its approval, Viagra has transformed the lives of countless men, restoring not only their sexual performance but also their confidence and emotional well-being. With decades of use and millions of prescriptions worldwide, Viagra remains one of the most reliable solutions for ED.

In the next chapter, we'll delve into the specific benefits of Viagra and why it continues to be a trusted option for men seeking to improve their sexual health.

Chapter 3: The Key Benefits of Viagra (Sildenafil)

Viagra (Sildenafil) is not just about solving a physical issue—it has a profound impact on overall sexual health and well-being. In this chapter, we'll explore the major benefits of using Viagra, beyond just achieving an erection, and why so many men continue to rely on it to enhance their sexual performance and confidence.

1. Stronger, Longer-Lasting Erections

One of the primary benefits of Viagra is its ability to help men achieve stronger, more reliable erections. Erectile dysfunction often results in erections that are either weak or difficult to maintain for the duration of sexual activity. With Viagra, men experience enhanced blood flow to the penis, allowing them to achieve firmer erections that last long enough for satisfying intercourse.

- **Improved Blood Circulation**: Viagra works by relaxing the smooth muscles in the blood vessels, allowing for increased blood flow to the erectile tissues in the penis. This enhanced circulation is what makes erections firmer and easier to maintain.

- **Duration of Effectiveness**: Once Viagra begins working, it can last for several hours, allowing men to enjoy spontaneous sexual experiences. Many men appreciate the fact that they don't have to rush into sexual activity or worry about losing their erection too quickly.

2. Quick and Reliable Results

Viagra is known for its fast-acting nature and its reliability, making it an excellent option for men who want a dependable solution to their erectile problems. Typically, Viagra starts working within 30 to 60 minutes after ingestion, which means that men can plan sexual activity without a long wait time.

- **Predictable Onset**: One of the advantages of Viagra is its predictable onset. As long as it's taken on an empty stomach or with a light meal, you can expect the medication to start working within the specified time frame. This predictability helps men feel more in control of their sexual performance.
- **Flexibility for Spontaneity**: With its effects lasting up to 4-5 hours, Viagra provides a window of time for intimacy. This allows for more flexibility in timing sexual encounters, reducing the stress or pressure that some men feel when trying to plan for sex.

3. Enhanced Sexual Confidence

The psychological benefits of Viagra are just as important as the physical ones. Many men who struggle with ED experience a loss of confidence in their sexual abilities, which can lead to performance anxiety, avoidance of intimacy, and even relationship problems. By restoring erectile function, Viagra plays a crucial role in rebuilding self-confidence in sexual situations.

- **Boost in Self-Esteem**: Men who regain their ability to perform sexually often report a significant boost in self-esteem. Knowing that you can rely on your body to perform can alleviate the anxiety and stress that often accompany ED.
- **Eliminating Fear of Failure**: Viagra reduces the fear of underperformance, which can be a major obstacle to sexual satisfaction. When you're confident that your body will respond, you can focus more on enjoying the moment and connecting with your partner.

4. Proven Solution for Erectile Dysfunction

Viagra is backed by years of research and clinical trials, making it one of the most trusted medications for treating ED. Its safety and efficacy have been demonstrated in numerous studies involving men of various ages and health conditions. This long-standing track record provides peace of mind for those considering Viagra as a solution.

- **Clinical Efficacy**: Research consistently shows that Viagra works for the majority of men who use it, regardless of the underlying cause of their ED. Whether the issue is physical (due to diabetes, cardiovascular disease, etc.) or psychological (due to stress or anxiety), Viagra has proven to be effective in most cases.
- **Approved by Health Authorities**: Viagra is FDA-approved and has been available for over two decades, which underscores its safety when used as directed. Over the years, millions of prescriptions have been filled worldwide, making it a cornerstone in the treatment of ED.

5. Restored Intimacy and Connection

Erectile dysfunction can take a significant toll on intimate relationships. When sexual performance becomes inconsistent or impossible, it often leads to frustration, tension, and emotional distance between partners. One of the most powerful benefits of Viagra is its ability to restore intimacy and rekindle the connection between partners.

- **Improved Relationship Satisfaction**: By addressing the physical challenges of ED, Viagra helps men re-establish physical intimacy, which often improves emotional closeness with their partners. When the pressure of sexual performance is removed, couples can focus on enjoying each other's company and strengthening their bond.
- **Reducing Tension**: Many couples experience stress and frustration when ED becomes a frequent issue. Viagra can help alleviate this tension, allowing for more relaxed and fulfilling sexual experiences. When both partners feel satisfied, it can lead to better communication and overall relationship harmony.

6. Benefits for Overall Well-Being

Though Viagra is primarily used for erectile dysfunction, its impact often extends to a man's overall well-being. Sexual health is a vital aspect of general health, and when this is improved, other areas of life often follow suit.

- **Better Mental Health**: Restoring sexual function can reduce feelings of depression, anxiety, and frustration. Many men find that overcoming ED improves their mood and reduces the stress that had built up around their inability to perform.

- **Greater Quality of Life**: Feeling confident in your ability to engage in intimate relationships can enhance your overall quality of life. Men often report feeling more satisfied, not just in the bedroom but in their daily lives, once the burden of ED is lifted.

Why Viagra Remains the Top Choice

With so many benefits, it's clear why Viagra remains one of the top choices for men seeking a solution to ED. The combination of its physical, psychological, and relationship-enhancing effects makes it an invaluable tool for men facing sexual challenges. It is not just a pill for achieving erections—it's a way to restore balance, connection, and confidence in your intimate life.

- **Trusted by Millions**: Over 20 million men have used Viagra, and its success stories are a testament to its transformative impact. Whether it's giving a man back his sexual prowess or helping him rebuild a connection with his partner, Viagra has been the go-to solution for more than two decades.
- **Accessible and Convenient**: Viagra's widespread availability and ease of use (an oral pill) make it a convenient option for men. With proper medical guidance, men can easily integrate it into their lives to enjoy consistent and reliable results.

Is Viagra Right for You?

While Viagra offers many benefits, it's important to remember that it's not suitable for everyone. Consulting with a healthcare provider is essential to determine if Viagra is the right treatment for your specific needs. A doctor can evaluate your overall health, any medications you're currently taking, and your specific symptoms to ensure that Viagra is safe and effective for you.

Chapter 4: Safety Considerations and Side Effects of Viagra (Sildenafil)

While Viagra (Sildenafil) is a highly effective solution for erectile dysfunction (ED), it is important to understand the safety guidelines and potential side effects associated with its use. Like all medications, Viagra can have side effects, and it is crucial to use it responsibly to ensure both its effectiveness and your overall well-being. In this chapter, we will cover the common and rare side effects of Viagra, its interactions with other medications, and how to use it safely.

1. Common Side Effects of Viagra

Most men who use Viagra experience few, if any, side effects. When side effects do occur, they are typically mild and temporary. Some of the most common side effects include:

- **Headache**: This is one of the most frequently reported side effects of Viagra. It occurs because the medication increases blood flow, which can also affect the blood vessels in the brain. The headache is usually mild and subsides as the medication wears off.

- **Flushing**: A feeling of warmth or redness, particularly in the face, neck, or chest, is another common side effect. Flushing occurs due to increased blood flow near the surface of the skin. It is usually harmless and temporary.
- **Nasal Congestion**: Some men may experience a stuffy nose after taking Viagra. This occurs because the drug affects blood flow in the nasal passages as well. Like other side effects, nasal congestion typically goes away on its own.
- **Indigestion or Upset Stomach**: Viagra can sometimes cause digestive discomfort, such as acid reflux or a mild upset stomach. Taking the medication with a light meal or avoiding heavy, fatty foods before taking Viagra can help minimize this effect.
- **Dizziness**: A small number of men may experience dizziness or lightheadedness after taking Viagra. This is due to the way the medication affects blood pressure. It is important to avoid sudden movements or standing up too quickly if you feel dizzy after taking Viagra.

2. Less Common Side Effects

Though less frequent, some men may experience the following side effects when taking Viagra:

- **Blurred Vision or Changes in Color Perception**: Viagra can sometimes cause temporary changes in vision, including blurriness or difficulty distinguishing between certain colors, particularly blue and green. These effects are rare and typically resolve on their own.
- **Muscle or Back Pain**: In rare cases, some men report experiencing muscle pain or back pain after taking Viagra. This can be uncomfortable but usually subsides within a few hours or days.
- **Prolonged Erection (Priapism)**: One of the more serious, though rare, side effects is priapism, which is an erection that lasts for more than four hours. If left untreated, priapism can cause permanent damage to the penis. If you experience an erection that lasts longer than four hours, it is important to seek immediate medical attention.

3. Rare but Serious Side Effects

While serious side effects from Viagra are uncommon, they can occur in some individuals. It's important to be aware of these risks and to contact a healthcare professional if you experience any of the following:

- **Severe Vision Loss**: In very rare cases, Viagra has been associated with a condition called **non-arteritic anterior ischemic optic neuropathy (NAION)**, which can lead to sudden vision loss in one or both eyes. If you experience any sudden changes in your vision, stop taking Viagra and seek medical help immediately.
- **Hearing Loss**: Another rare side effect of Viagra is sudden hearing loss or ringing in the ears. If you notice any changes in your hearing, discontinue use and contact your doctor right away.
- **Severe Allergic Reactions**: In extremely rare cases, men may have an allergic reaction to Viagra. Symptoms can include swelling of the face, lips, or throat, difficulty breathing, or a rash. If you suspect an allergic reaction, seek emergency medical care immediately.

4. Who Should Not Take Viagra?

While Viagra is safe for most men, there are certain individuals who should avoid using it or who should use it only under strict medical supervision. If any of the following applies to you, it's essential to consult your doctor before taking Viagra:

- **Men Taking Nitrates**: Viagra should never be used by men who are taking nitrates for heart conditions, such as nitroglycerin, isosorbide mononitrate, or isosorbide dinitrate. Nitrates and Viagra both lower blood pressure, and taking them together can cause a dangerous drop in blood pressure, leading to fainting, heart attack, or stroke.
- **Men with Severe Heart or Liver Problems**: If you have a serious heart condition, such as severe heart disease or congestive heart failure, or significant liver impairment, Viagra may not be safe for you. In such cases, your doctor will need to evaluate your condition to determine if you can take the medication.
- **Men with Hypotension or Uncontrolled Hypertension**: Men with extremely low blood pressure (hypotension) or uncontrolled high blood pressure (hypertension) should avoid taking Viagra. Your doctor may recommend an alternative treatment or adjust your current medications to make Viagra safer for use.

- **Men with Certain Eye Conditions**: If you have a history of certain eye conditions, such as retinitis pigmentosa or NAION, you may be at higher risk for vision-related side effects from Viagra. Discuss your medical history with your doctor to assess whether Viagra is appropriate for you.

5. Medication Interactions

Viagra can interact with other medications, which may either enhance or diminish its effects. It's important to tell your doctor about all the medications and supplements you are taking before starting Viagra, including:

- **Blood Pressure Medications**: Viagra can lower blood pressure, so if you are already taking medication for hypertension, your doctor may need to adjust your dosage or recommend an alternative ED treatment.
- **Alpha-Blockers**: Used to treat prostate enlargement or high blood pressure, alpha-blockers can interact with Viagra and cause a significant drop in blood pressure, leading to dizziness or fainting.
- **Other ED Medications**: Never take Viagra alongside other medications for ED, such as Cialis (tadalafil) or Levitra (vardenafil), as this can increase the risk of side effects without improving effectiveness.

- **Antifungal or Antibiotic Medications**:
  Certain antifungal drugs (like
  ketoconazole) or antibiotics (like
  erythromycin) can interfere with the
  metabolism of Viagra, causing it to
  remain in the body longer and potentially
  increasing the risk of side effects.

6. How to Use Viagra Safely

To ensure that Viagra is both safe and effective,
follow these guidelines:

- **Take Only the Prescribed Dose**: Viagra is
  available in various doses (25 mg, 50 mg,
  100 mg). Your doctor will recommend the
  appropriate dose based on your health
  and the severity of your ED. Never take
  more than one dose in a 24-hour period,
  and avoid increasing the dose on your
  own.
- **Avoid Alcohol and High-Fat Meals**:
  While moderate alcohol consumption is
  generally safe, excessive drinking can
  interfere with your ability to achieve an
  erection and may increase the risk of side
  effects. Additionally, high-fat meals can
  delay the absorption of Viagra, making it
  less effective. For best results, take Viagra
  on an empty stomach or after a light meal.

- **Monitor Your Body's Response**: Pay attention to how your body reacts to Viagra. If you experience any unusual symptoms or side effects, stop taking the medication and consult your doctor. Regular follow-ups with your healthcare provider can help adjust your treatment as needed.
- **Don't Combine with Recreational Drugs**: The use of recreational drugs, particularly "poppers" (amyl nitrite or butyl nitrite), in combination with Viagra is extremely dangerous and can lead to serious health complications.

7. When to Seek Medical Help

If you experience any of the following while taking Viagra, seek immediate medical attention:

- Chest pain, shortness of breath, or dizziness
- A prolonged erection lasting more than 4 hours
- Sudden vision or hearing loss
- Severe allergic reaction (rash, swelling, difficulty breathing)

Conclusion: Safe Use is Key

Viagra has been a game-changer for millions of men, allowing them to overcome erectile dysfunction and regain their sexual confidence. However, like all medications, it should be used responsibly. By understanding the potential side effects, knowing how to use it safely, and consulting your doctor about any concerns, you can maximize the benefits of Viagra while minimizing the risks.

In the next chapter, we'll explore the emotional and psychological benefits of Viagra, and how addressing ED can improve not just sexual performance, but also your mental and emotional well-being.

Chapter 5: Emotional and Psychological Benefits of Viagra (Sildenafil)

While Viagra (Sildenafil) is primarily known for its physical effects — helping men achieve and maintain erections — its emotional and psychological benefits are equally important. Erectile dysfunction (ED) often has a profound impact on a man's mental health, self-esteem, and relationships. In this chapter, we'll explore how Viagra can improve more than just your sexual performance, offering a renewed sense of confidence, emotional well-being, and connection with your partner.

1. Restoring Self-Confidence

One of the most immediate emotional benefits of Viagra is the restoration of self-confidence. For men suffering from ED, the inability to perform sexually can lead to feelings of inadequacy, embarrassment, and frustration. Over time, this can erode a man's self-esteem, making him hesitant to engage in intimate situations or even avoid them altogether.

- **The Confidence to Perform**: By addressing the physical issue of ED, Viagra helps eliminate the fear of failure that many men experience. Knowing that they have a reliable way to achieve an erection can significantly boost self-assurance, making men feel more in control of their sexual performance.

- **Overcoming Anxiety**: Performance anxiety is a common problem for men with ED. The worry that they won't be able to perform can create a vicious cycle, where anxiety worsens their ability to get or maintain an erection. Viagra helps break this cycle by providing a dependable solution, allowing men to focus on the moment rather than worrying about whether their body will cooperate.
- **Improving Body Image**: ED can sometimes make men feel disconnected from their own bodies, leading to negative body image or self-consciousness about their masculinity. By restoring sexual function, Viagra can help men feel more in tune with their physical selves, improving their overall self-image and sense of masculinity.

2. Reducing Stress and Depression

The emotional toll of ED often extends beyond the bedroom. Many men with ED report experiencing higher levels of stress and depression, particularly if the condition persists over time. Sexual performance is closely tied to identity and self-worth for many men, and ongoing difficulties in this area can contribute to a range of mental health challenges.

- **Alleviating the Emotional Burden**: Viagra helps alleviate the stress associated with ED by offering a consistent solution. Men who no longer have to worry about their sexual performance may find that their overall stress levels decrease, leading to improvements in their mental and emotional health.
- **Improving Mood**: Sexual satisfaction and intimacy are linked to the release of endorphins and other mood-enhancing chemicals in the brain. When ED prevents a man from enjoying these experiences, it can negatively impact his mood and contribute to feelings of sadness or frustration. By helping men regain their sexual function, Viagra indirectly supports better mental health by enabling more fulfilling intimate experiences.
- **Combating Isolation**: Many men with ED avoid discussing their condition out of embarrassment or shame. This can lead to isolation, both emotionally and socially. By addressing the root cause of ED, Viagra gives men the confidence to re-engage in social and romantic activities, reducing feelings of loneliness or isolation.

3. Rebuilding Intimacy in Relationships

Erectile dysfunction doesn't just affect the man experiencing it—it also has a profound impact on his partner and their relationship. When sexual performance becomes inconsistent or unreliable, it often leads to tension, frustration, and emotional distance between partners. Viagra can play a vital role in rebuilding intimacy and connection by restoring sexual function and improving communication between partners.

- **Restoring Physical Intimacy**: For many couples, physical intimacy is an important part of maintaining a strong emotional bond. ED can disrupt this, leading to a decrease in sexual activity and closeness. By helping men regain their ability to perform sexually, Viagra allows couples to rediscover the pleasure of physical intimacy, which can help strengthen their overall relationship.

- **Improving Emotional Communication**: The emotional challenges associated with ED often lead to communication breakdowns between partners. Men may avoid discussing their struggles out of embarrassment, while their partners may feel rejected or unsure of how to help. When Viagra effectively treats ED, it can open the door to more honest and supportive communication, as both partners feel more secure in their relationship.

- **Reducing Relationship Tension**: Sexual difficulties can be a major source of tension in relationships, often leading to frustration or misunderstandings. Partners may misinterpret ED as a sign of disinterest or infidelity, further straining the relationship. Viagra helps alleviate this tension by addressing the root cause of the problem, allowing couples to focus on rebuilding their emotional and physical connection.

4. Enhancing Overall Relationship Satisfaction

Sexual satisfaction is a key component of relationship satisfaction for many couples. When sexual difficulties like ED are resolved, it often leads to greater happiness and harmony in the relationship as a whole. Viagra not only improves sexual performance but also enhances the quality of life by restoring an important aspect of intimacy.

- **Renewed Passion**: For couples who have struggled with ED, the return of consistent sexual performance can reignite the passion in their relationship. Viagra provides the opportunity to enjoy spontaneous, fulfilling sexual experiences once again, which can renew the excitement and romance between partners.

- **Boosting Trust and Security**: ED can sometimes lead to feelings of insecurity or mistrust within a relationship. When sexual performance is unreliable, partners may begin to feel uncertain about the stability of their relationship. By offering a dependable solution to ED, Viagra can help restore trust and a sense of security, allowing both partners to feel more confident in their relationship.

5. Addressing the Stigma Around ED

One of the psychological challenges associated with ED is the stigma surrounding it. Many men feel ashamed to admit that they are struggling with ED, which can prevent them from seeking help. Viagra not only provides a physical solution but also helps break down the barriers of silence and embarrassment around ED.

- **Normalizing the Conversation**: As more men become open about their experiences with ED and the benefits of using Viagra, it helps reduce the stigma attached to the condition. By discussing ED openly and honestly, men can feel less isolated and more empowered to take control of their sexual health.

- **Encouraging Medical Consultation**: For many men, the decision to seek treatment for ED can be difficult due to feelings of embarrassment or denial. Knowing that there is a well-established and effective treatment like Viagra can encourage men to speak with their healthcare providers and take proactive steps to improve their sexual health.

6. Viagra's Role in Improving Quality of Life

Ultimately, the emotional and psychological benefits of Viagra extend far beyond the bedroom. For many men, addressing ED leads to improvements in their overall quality of life. When men feel confident in their ability to perform sexually, they often experience greater satisfaction in other areas of life, including their relationships, social interactions, and mental well-being.

- **Restoring a Sense of Control**: ED can make men feel as though they've lost control over an important aspect of their lives. By restoring sexual function, Viagra helps men regain control, which boosts their confidence and reduces feelings of helplessness or frustration.

- **Improving General Well-Being**: A fulfilling sex life is an important aspect of overall health and well-being. By addressing ED, Viagra contributes to a more balanced and satisfying life, allowing men to enjoy a higher level of emotional and physical health.

Conclusion: A Holistic Impact

While Viagra's most immediate effect is physical, its emotional and psychological benefits are just as significant. From restoring self-confidence and alleviating stress to rebuilding intimacy and improving relationship satisfaction, Viagra can have a transformative impact on a man's life. By addressing both the physical and emotional aspects of erectile dysfunction, Viagra offers men a chance to reclaim their sense of self and experience a renewed sense of joy and connection in their relationships.

In the next chapter, we'll explore how men can make informed decisions about using Viagra, including the importance of consulting a healthcare professional and understanding the available options.

Chapter 6: Making an Informed Decision About Viagra (Sildenafil)

Deciding whether to take Viagra (Sildenafil) for erectile dysfunction (ED) is an important step toward improving your sexual health and overall well-being. However, it's essential to approach this decision thoughtfully and with all the necessary information. In this chapter, we'll explore the factors you should consider when deciding whether Viagra is right for you, how to consult with a healthcare provider, and the available options for purchasing the medication.

1. Understanding Your Condition

Before deciding on a treatment like Viagra, it's crucial to understand the root cause of your erectile dysfunction. ED can have both physical and psychological causes, and the most effective treatment plan may vary depending on your individual circumstances.

- **Physical Causes**: ED is often linked to underlying health conditions such as diabetes, heart disease, high blood pressure, obesity, or hormonal imbalances. If your ED is related to these issues, addressing the underlying health problems may be part of the overall treatment plan. Viagra can help manage ED, but it's also important to work on improving your overall health.

- **Psychological Causes**: Stress, anxiety, depression, and relationship problems are common psychological causes of ED. In cases where mental health plays a significant role, counseling or therapy, combined with Viagra, can be an effective solution. Understanding whether your ED is primarily psychological or physical will help guide your decision-making process.
- **Age-Related Factors**: While ED can occur at any age, it becomes more common as men get older. Age-related ED is often due to reduced blood flow and changes in vascular health. Viagra is particularly effective for men whose ED is linked to these age-related changes, making it a viable option for men in their 40s, 50s, and beyond.

2. Consulting a Healthcare Provider

Viagra is a prescription medication, which means it's important to consult with a healthcare provider before starting treatment. Your doctor will assess your overall health, the severity of your ED, and any other medications or conditions that could affect your treatment. Here's what you can expect during your consultation:

- **Medical History Review**: Your doctor will ask about your medical history, including any chronic health conditions, surgeries, or medications you are currently taking. This is important because certain conditions, such as heart disease or high blood pressure, may affect whether Viagra is safe for you.
- **Physical Examination**: In some cases, your doctor may perform a physical examination to check your cardiovascular health, blood pressure, and overall fitness. Since ED can sometimes be an early warning sign of cardiovascular problems, your doctor may want to rule out any serious underlying conditions.
- **Discussion of Symptoms**: Be prepared to discuss your symptoms in detail, including how often you experience ED, whether you can achieve erections during non-sexual situations (such as during sleep), and any other factors that may be affecting your sexual health. This information helps your doctor understand the severity and causes of your ED.

- **Prescription and Dosage**: If your doctor determines that Viagra is suitable for you, they will prescribe the appropriate dosage. Viagra is available in doses of 25 mg, 50 mg, and 100 mg. Your doctor will likely start you on a moderate dose and adjust it based on how well the medication works and whether you experience any side effects.

3. Weighing the Benefits and Risks

As with any medication, it's important to weigh the benefits of Viagra against the potential risks or side effects. Understanding both will help you make an informed decision about whether Viagra is right for you.

- **Benefits**: Viagra has a proven track record of helping men achieve stronger, longer-lasting erections. It offers a quick, reliable solution to ED, which can improve confidence, relationship satisfaction, and overall quality of life. For many men, the emotional and psychological benefits are just as valuable as the physical effects.

- **Risks**: As discussed in the previous chapter, Viagra can cause mild side effects such as headaches, flushing, and indigestion. More serious risks, such as priapism (prolonged erections) or sudden vision loss, are rare but possible. Additionally, if you have certain medical conditions, such as heart disease or take medications like nitrates, Viagra may not be safe for you.

By discussing the risks and benefits with your healthcare provider, you can make a decision that balances the improvement in your sexual health with your overall safety.

4. Generic vs. Brand Name: Understanding Your Options

When it comes to purchasing Viagra, you have two main options: the brand-name version of Viagra or its generic counterpart, Sildenafil. Both options are effective, but there are some differences in cost, availability, and branding that you should consider.

- **Brand Name Viagra**: Viagra was developed and patented by Pfizer and has been on the market since 1998. Many men prefer the brand-name version because of its strong reputation and long history of success. However, it tends to be more expensive than generic options.

- **Generic Sildenafil**: After Pfizer's patent on Viagra expired, generic versions of Sildenafil became widely available. These generics are just as effective as brand-name Viagra, as they contain the same active ingredient. The primary difference is the price — generic Sildenafil is usually much cheaper, making it a more affordable option for long-term use.
- **Choosing Between the Two**: For most men, the choice between brand-name Viagra and generic Sildenafil comes down to cost. If the price of Viagra is a concern, opting for the generic version can offer the same benefits at a fraction of the price. However, some men may feel more comfortable sticking with the brand name due to its established reputation. Either option should be discussed with your healthcare provider.

5. How to Buy Viagra Safely

Once you have a prescription, it's important to ensure you are purchasing Viagra from a reputable source. Unfortunately, the market is flooded with counterfeit or low-quality versions of ED medications, especially online. To ensure your safety, follow these guidelines when buying Viagra:

- **Buy from a Licensed Pharmacy**: Always purchase Viagra from a licensed pharmacy, whether it's an in-person location or an online service. Licensed pharmacies will require a prescription and provide the genuine product. Be wary of websites or sellers that offer Viagra without a prescription—this is a major red flag.
- **Avoid Counterfeit Products**: Counterfeit Viagra is a significant problem, particularly online. These fake medications may not contain the active ingredient Sildenafil or could contain harmful substances. Stick to well-known, legitimate pharmacies, and avoid buying Viagra from dubious or unverified sources.
- **Consider Telemedicine Services**: In recent years, telemedicine platforms have made it easier to consult with a doctor and get a prescription for Viagra without needing to visit a physical office. These services typically offer a simple online consultation with a licensed physician, who can prescribe Viagra if appropriate. Many telemedicine services also ship the medication directly to your home, offering convenience and discretion.

6. The Role of Lifestyle Changes

While Viagra is an effective treatment for ED, it's important to remember that lifestyle factors also play a crucial role in sexual health. Making positive changes in your daily habits can improve the effectiveness of Viagra and even reduce the severity of ED over time.

- **Exercise Regularly**: Physical activity is one of the best ways to improve blood flow, cardiovascular health, and overall fitness — all of which can help with erectile function. Regular exercise can also reduce stress and boost mood, further enhancing your sexual performance.
- **Maintain a Healthy Diet**: A balanced diet that is rich in fruits, vegetables, whole grains, and lean proteins can support better heart health and circulation. Avoiding excessive amounts of processed foods, high-fat meals, and sugary snacks can improve both your overall health and your sexual health.
- **Manage Stress**: Chronic stress can have a negative impact on sexual performance and may contribute to ED. Practice stress management techniques such as mindfulness, meditation, yoga, or other relaxation methods to reduce stress and anxiety in your life.

- **Limit Alcohol and Tobacco**: Excessive alcohol consumption and smoking are major risk factors for ED. Reducing or eliminating these substances can improve blood flow and reduce the severity of ED, making Viagra more effective.

7. Alternatives to Viagra

Viagra is not the only treatment option for erectile dysfunction. Depending on your health condition, preferences, and response to treatment, your doctor may suggest alternatives such as:

- **Other ED Medications**: Cialis (tadalafil) and Levitra (vardenafil) are two other commonly prescribed medications for ED. These drugs work similarly to Viagra but have different durations of action and onset times. For example, Cialis can last up to 36 hours, offering more flexibility for spontaneous sexual activity.
- **Vacuum Erection Devices**: These mechanical devices use a vacuum to draw blood into the penis, creating an erection. While they may not be as convenient as medication, they can be a good option for men who cannot take oral medications for ED.

- **Penile Injections**: In some cases, doctors may recommend injecting medication directly into the penis to produce an erection. This method is highly effective, but it requires training and a certain level of comfort with self-injection.
- **Counseling or Therapy**: If your ED has psychological causes, working with a therapist can help address underlying issues such as anxiety, depression, or relationship problems. Therapy can be especially helpful when combined with medications like Viagra.

Conclusion: Making the Right Choice for You

Choosing whether to take Viagra and how to incorporate it into your treatment plan is a highly personal decision. By understanding your condition, consulting with a healthcare provider, and considering your options, you can make an informed choice that is right for you. Viagra offers a reliable and proven solution for many men, but it's important to use it as part of a holistic approach to sexual health that includes lifestyle changes and open communication with your partner and healthcare provider.

In the next chapter, we'll share real-life success stories from men who have used Viagra to improve their sexual health and relationships, offering inspiration and insight into how this medication can make a positive difference.

Chapter 7: Real-Life Success Stories
The effectiveness of Viagra (Sildenafil) goes beyond just clinical data and studies. For many men, Viagra has been a life-changing solution, not only restoring sexual function but also improving self-esteem, relationships, and overall happiness. In this chapter, we'll share real-life stories from men who have successfully used Viagra to overcome erectile dysfunction (ED) and reclaim control over their intimate lives. These personal accounts offer insight into the transformative impact of Viagra and highlight the emotional, psychological, and relational benefits it can bring.

1. David's Story: A Return to Confidence
David, a 52-year-old man, had been struggling with ED for a few years. His problem started gradually but eventually became so severe that he was unable to maintain an erection. The loss of sexual function deeply affected his self-confidence, and he found himself avoiding intimate situations with his wife out of fear of failure.

- **The Strain on His Relationship**: "I felt like I was letting my wife down, even though she was incredibly understanding. It wasn't just about the sex; it was about the closeness and connection that we were losing. I started to feel like a shadow of myself, and it took a toll on my confidence in all areas of my life."
- **Finding a Solution**: After discussing his problem with his doctor, David was prescribed Viagra. He was nervous at first, but after his first experience with the medication, he quickly saw how effective it was. "It was a game changer for me. Within about 45 minutes, I could feel the difference. The confidence came flooding back."
- **Rebuilding Intimacy**: Viagra not only restored David's ability to perform sexually but also helped rebuild the emotional intimacy between him and his wife. "The emotional distance that had developed between us melted away. We were able to reconnect on a deeper level, and the confidence I gained extended to other areas of my life as well."

David's story highlights how Viagra can do more than improve sexual performance—it can restore the emotional closeness in a relationship and boost a man's overall sense of self-worth.

2. Mark's Story: Overcoming Anxiety and Stress

Mark, a 38-year-old professional, had experienced occasional bouts of ED, particularly during stressful periods in his life. While his ED was not constant, it became a source of anxiety, making him worry about his ability to perform sexually, especially with new partners.

- **The Vicious Cycle of Anxiety**: "For me, it wasn't so much a physical issue as it was mental. I'd get anxious about whether I'd be able to perform, and that anxiety would actually prevent me from getting an erection. It became a self-fulfilling prophecy."
- **Breaking the Cycle with Viagra**: Mark turned to Viagra after discussing his concerns with his doctor. "Viagra helped break that cycle of anxiety. Knowing I had a reliable solution took a huge weight off my shoulders. I didn't have to worry about whether I'd be able to perform, which meant I could actually relax and enjoy the moment."

- **Building Confidence in New Relationships**: Mark found that Viagra not only addressed his physical symptoms but also helped him feel more secure and confident in intimate situations. "It gave me the confidence to be present and connect with my partner, without the constant worry in the back of my mind. That made a huge difference in my dating life."

Mark's story demonstrates how Viagra can alleviate the psychological pressures associated with ED, allowing men to enjoy sex without the looming fear of underperformance.

3. Carlos' Story: Rediscovering Passion After Heart Surgery

Carlos, a 60-year-old man, had undergone heart surgery and was on several medications for high blood pressure. While the surgery had saved his life, it had also led to problems with erectile function, and he wasn't sure if there was a safe solution for him.

- **Concerns About Safety**: "After my surgery, I was worried about taking any kind of medication for ED. I didn't want to do anything that might put my heart at risk. But at the same time, I was missing the intimacy I used to have with my wife. We had always had a very passionate relationship, and I didn't want to lose that."

- **Consulting His Doctor**: Carlos consulted his cardiologist, who reassured him that Viagra could be used safely, as long as it wasn't combined with nitrates. "My doctor explained how Viagra worked and how it could actually be a safe option for me. We worked together to adjust my medications, and I felt comfortable trying it out."
- **A Renewed Relationship**: After starting on Viagra, Carlos and his wife were able to rekindle their physical intimacy. "It was like getting a part of our marriage back. We felt closer, and it reminded us of how important that part of our relationship was. Viagra gave us that spark again, and it's made a huge difference in how we relate to each other."

Carlos' story emphasizes the importance of consulting a healthcare provider when considering Viagra, especially for men with heart conditions. With the right guidance, men can safely enjoy the benefits of Viagra without compromising their health.

4. James' Story: Finding Hope After Years of Struggle

James, a 45-year-old man, had been living with ED for nearly five years before he decided to seek help. For James, ED had become a source of shame, and he avoided discussing it, even with his doctor. Over time, this avoidance took a toll on his marriage and his mental health.

- **Feeling Isolated**: "I didn't want to admit that I had a problem. I thought it was something I should be able to fix on my own, but the more I ignored it, the worse it got. I started to withdraw from my wife, and it made me feel really isolated."
- **Taking the First Step**: After some encouragement from his wife, James finally opened up to his doctor, who prescribed Viagra. "It was hard to talk about at first, but once I got over that initial hurdle, it felt like a weight had been lifted. My doctor was very understanding, and I realized that I wasn't alone—ED is more common than I thought."

- **Rebuilding His Confidence**: After trying Viagra, James found that it not only solved his physical problem but also helped him reconnect with his wife on an emotional level. "Viagra gave me back the ability to perform, but more than that, it helped me feel confident again. My wife and I were able to rebuild our relationship, and I stopped feeling like I was hiding this secret."

James' story is a powerful example of how seeking help can make a world of difference. For men who feel isolated or ashamed of their ED, taking that first step toward treatment can be life-changing, both physically and emotionally.

5. Tom's Story: A Second Chance After Prostate Surgery

Tom, a 62-year-old man, had undergone prostate surgery for cancer, which left him dealing with ED. While the surgery was successful in treating his cancer, the resulting ED deeply affected his self-esteem and his relationship with his wife.

- **Post-Surgery Struggles**: "I knew going into the surgery that ED might be a side effect, but it was still hard to deal with afterward. I didn't feel like myself anymore, and I didn't know if I'd ever be able to have a normal sex life again."

- **A Solution with Viagra**: After his recovery, Tom's doctor suggested trying Viagra to see if it could help restore his sexual function. "At first, I wasn't sure if it would work, but I figured it was worth a try. I was amazed at how well it worked. It didn't just give me back my sexual function — it gave me back a sense of normalcy."
- **Reclaiming Intimacy**: For Tom and his wife, Viagra helped them reconnect after a difficult period. "It wasn't just about the physical side — it was about feeling like we were getting our relationship back. We could be intimate again, and that brought us closer together emotionally."

Tom's story highlights how Viagra can provide a second chance at intimacy after medical procedures like prostate surgery. It offers hope to men who may feel that their sexual health has been permanently affected by illness or surgery.

Conclusion: The Power of Viagra in Real Life

These real-life stories demonstrate the profound impact that Viagra can have on men's lives, helping them overcome the physical and emotional challenges of erectile dysfunction. Whether dealing with age-related ED, anxiety, or the aftermath of medical procedures, Viagra offers a reliable solution that can restore confidence, rebuild relationships, and improve overall quality of life.

By sharing these stories, we hope to inspire men who are struggling with ED to seek help and explore the options available to them. Viagra has been a transformative solution for millions of men, and with the right guidance and support, it can help you regain control of your sexual health and experience the satisfaction and confidence you deserve.

Conclusion: Take Charge of Your Sexual Health

Erectile dysfunction can feel overwhelming, but it doesn't have to define you. Through this guide, we've explored how Viagra (Sildenafil) offers a reliable and proven solution for millions of men worldwide. Whether you're dealing with physical causes like cardiovascular issues or psychological factors such as stress and anxiety, Viagra has the potential to restore your confidence, intimacy, and overall quality of life. Key takeaways from this guide include:

- **Understanding ED**: Knowing the underlying causes of ED can help you and your healthcare provider choose the most effective treatment approach.
- **How Viagra Works**: By improving blood flow to the penis, Viagra helps men achieve and maintain strong, lasting erections, offering quick and reliable results.
- **Safety First**: While Viagra is generally safe for most men, it's important to use it responsibly and consult a healthcare provider to determine if it's right for you.
- **Emotional and Relationship Benefits**: Beyond the physical effects, Viagra can restore self-confidence, reduce anxiety, and improve relationship satisfaction by helping you reconnect with your partner.

- **Informed Decisions**: Whether choosing between brand-name Viagra or its generic counterpart, Sildenafil, or exploring lifestyle changes to complement your treatment, being informed is key to maximizing the benefits of Viagra.

Take the Next Step

If you're struggling with ED, know that you're not alone, and solutions like Viagra are readily available to help. By consulting with your healthcare provider and making informed choices, you can regain control of your sexual health and experience the emotional and relational benefits that come with it.

Don't let erectile dysfunction hold you back any longer. Take charge of your health, explore your options, and reclaim your confidence and vitality with the proven power of Viagra. The journey to a fulfilling and satisfying intimate life starts today.

Notes & Personal Reflections

This section is designed for you to reflect on your own experiences, keep track of your thoughts, and note any questions or insights that arise as you explore your options with Viagra (Sildenafil) or other treatments for erectile dysfunction. Use this space to document your journey toward improved sexual health and well-being.

Questions for My Doctor:
- What dosage of Viagra is right for me?
- Are there any potential interactions with my current medications?
- What lifestyle changes could improve my erectile function?
- How should I address any side effects if they occur?

Goals for Improving Sexual Health:
- What are my main concerns about erectile dysfunction?
- How would I like my intimate relationships to improve?
- What lifestyle changes can I make to complement my treatment? (e.g., diet, exercise, stress management)

Personal Progress Tracker:
- Date when I started using Viagra:

- Notes about my experiences (e.g., how I felt, effectiveness of the medication, any side effects):

Reflections on My Relationship:
- How has my partner supported me in this journey?
- What are my goals for improving intimacy and communication in my relationship?

Additional Thoughts:
- Use this space to write down any other reflections, successes, or challenges you experience along the way.

Made in United States
Troutdale, OR
01/29/2025

28469230R00040